The Answer to Cancer – An Electron Deficit Condition

Published by SAGAX Publishing
www.keithfoster.co.uk

Copyright © Keith Foster – June 2016

ISBN 978-0-9532407-5-3

A catalogue record for this book is available from the British Library

Keith Foster's right to be identified as the author of this work has been asserted by him in accordance with the Copyright, Designs and
Patents Act of 1988.

Manufacture / Printing coordinated in the UK by LightningSource.com

All rights reserved. No part of this book may be reproduced or transmitted in any form, electronic or mechanical, including photocopy or any information storage and retrieval system, with permission in writing from the publisher.

The Answer to Cancer – An Electron Deficit Condition

This work is dedicated to my wife Paula
whom I have loved for 40 years.
"The best is yet to come".

Preface

One of the contributing factors in the current cancer epidemic is the huge change that has taken place in our environment.

The separation from the natural rhythms and potential charges that previously invigorated us has had a profound effect, and this reflects in our overall health.

We are now surrounded and immersed in strong electro-magnetic fields which challenge our living structure by placing unusual loads on it. (e.g. mobile phones). Whilst, at the same time, preventing the natural recharge systems in our bodies from performing their essential functions properly.

In this book I describe in detail humankind's electro-magnetic (and sonic) nature so that you, dear reader, can get a better idea of how our bodies work on an electro-magnetic level, and can take steps to improve your health naturally.

The basic mechanism involved is the provision and transportation of electrons into flagging cells of the body, in order to recharge their energy levels and bring them 'up to speed' again. Also, to provide an adequate supply of electrons to damp down the excess oxidative bursts, which may be occurring throughout the body, so as to reduce inflammation and pain.

This is not a rapid process and is mediated by other factors such as diet, environment and your present condition. However, by following the suggestions I make you can significantly improve your health.

As your health begins to improve, your immune system cuts fully in again and begins to clear up and attend to the bacterial debris attendant on the destruction of the cancer.

The Answer to Cancer – An Electron Deficit Condition

This is vital to the future integrity of your bloodstream and is assisted by the information I give on the use of natural herbs long used and recommended in this role.

For your convenience I provide a food list (pages 84 - 88) and since you would be wise to change your diet, the information in this list will help.

In Appendices 1 & 2, I provide the information that you will need to fully comprehend humankind's electro-magnetic environment, its history, the reason for its current collapse and the effect of this on your health.

The Answer to Cancer – An Electron Deficit Condition

Other titles by Keith Foster

Perfume, Astrology and You. ISBN 978-0-9532407-0-8

Lifelight – *(How to protect yourself from cancer or help yourself if you get ill).* ISBN 978-0-9532407-1-5

Catastrophe – A New Theory as to the Cause of Global Warming. ISBN 978-0-9532407-3-9

The Wisdom Way. ISBN 978-0-9532407-9-1

Harmonic Power Parts II – VI; ISBN 978-0-9532407-7-7

The Backball Method – A Comprehensive Self-Help Guide to Back Pain Relief. ISBN 978-0-9532407-2-2

> ### Disclaimer
> This publication is for information only and should not be used for the diagnosis or treatment of medical conditions. If you are ill or have a medical condition first consult a qualified doctor or specialist.

The Answer to Cancer – An Electron Deficit Condition

Contents

PART 1

10 - 22   **Chapter 1 – CANCER**
pH; Negative ions; The Mechanism; Red blood cells; Low frequency current; White blood cells; The Regulator; The Recharge system; Overkill; Summary; Vital life; Acidic waste.

23 - 33   **Chapter 2 – VITAMIN C**
This is how it works; Essential fatty acids; Conclusion; Recommendation (A); Water; Water & ageing; Recommendation (B); Chlorinated water; How to reduce your exposure to chlorine / fluorine.

34 - 48   **Chapter 3 – IODINE**
More on Vitamin C, Vitamin E & Selenium; Self and not self; Vitamin E; Selenium; Scurvy; How Much; Bioflavonoids.

49 - 53   **Chapter 4 – CHARCOAL**
Adsorption.

54 - 58   **Chapter 5 - Turmeric**
The trade-off; Anti-cancer activity.

59 - 66	**Chapter 6 - Alkalinity / acidity** Alkaline tide; Cooking; Vitamins and minerals; Sodium bicarbonate supplementation.
67 - 71	**Chapter 7 – FASTING – RESTRICTED DIET**
72 - 83	**Chapter 8 - Blood cleanse** Conclusion; Fasting; Final thoughts; My daily dosages; Cachexia.

PART 2

84 - 88	**Chapter 9 - pH Foods list.**

PART 3
Appendices 1 & 2

89 – 110	**Chapter 10 – How to Slow Down the Aging Process** Magnetism and Earthing; Magnetic Fields on Health; Decline; Diurnal Flow; Our new electronic environment; How to protect yourself; Earthing is dose related; Disconnecting; Blood thinning; Inflammation and Ageing; Magnetic field.

111 - 125	**Chapter 11 – How to Lengthen Your (Healthy) Life** The Human Antenna. Here's How; Ancient civilizations; Cro-Magnon; Iron; Magnetic lines of Force.
126 – 135	**Chapter 12 – Resonance and Harmonics** A coupled oscillator; To bring things to a head; Summary; Addendum.
136	Recommended reading list.
137 - 140	References

PART 1

Chapter 1

CANCER

There is no cure for cancer and there probably never will be! This is because cancer is a condition, not a disease.

You <u>can</u> recover from cancer if you reverse the condition and this book sets out the various ways that this could be achieved.

Let me be clear, I'm not offering a "cure" for cancer but am simply laying out a methodology (backed by scientific proof) by which you may help yourself and recover naturally. All the information I detail here is published elsewhere by some of the world's leading thinkers and researchers. However, the interpretation I place on their conclusions is my own, based on a lifetime of thought, research and my own experiences.

The Answer to Cancer – An Electron Deficit Condition

I'm now 75 years of age, in vigorous good health and possessed of a lively enquiring mind. I believe that I have made a breakthrough in understanding cancer and share this with you in the belief that this may help you.

Cancer cells are very similar to mould or fungi cells. They look similar under a microscope and they use fermentation as their energy source. They also respond to anti-fungal measures. However, according to leading Australian researcher Walter Last whose articles *"Is Invasive Cancer a Hyphal Fungus"* and *"The New Direction in Cancer Therapy"* are available online, there is one major difference between cancer cells and fungal cells:- cancerous cells can be revived, can be switched back to being healthy body cells again, whereas fungal cells cannot, they always remain fungal cells.

Cancer cells become cancerous when their energy levels are exhausted and the RNA "readout" mechanism, which forms part of the

DNA helix, is unable to obtain sufficient energy from the exhausted cell to respond normally and reverts to an earlier more primitive method of energy generation which is fermentation. Fermentation only produces about 5% of the energy that the cell normally produces in what's known as the citric acid cycle and fermentation generates large amounts of lactic acid which is basically unburnt glucose and which causes the body to become yet more acidic.

Acidity is at the very core of the cancerous process since cancer cannot exist in an alkaline environment. An alkaline environment is capable of absorbing significantly more oxygen than an acidic one and it is the oxygen content of the system which dictates the degree of cancer to which it is susceptible.

It was Dr. Otto Warburg MD, the greatest bio-chemist of the 20th century, who did all the ground breaking research into respiratory enzymes, vitamins and minerals that the body requires for the utilisation of oxygen in the cells.

This earned him the Nobel Prize in 1931 and he also discovered how to measure the pressure of oxygen in a living cell. This led to the discovery that low oxygen concentration and pressure always presages the development of cancer.

He clearly stated that the most basic cause of cancer is too little oxygen getting into the cell and he said "we find by experimentation about 35% inhibition of oxygen respiration already suffices to bring about such transformation during cell growth".

That's it! Just one third less oxygen than normal and you can contract cancer.

pH.

pH is the balance between acid and alkaline in any substance and human blood has a pH value ranging from 7.3 to 7.45. 7.45 contains 64.9% more excess oxygen than blood with a pH value of 7.3 and if the blood develops a more acidic condition, your body deposits these excess acidic substances in some area out of the way so that the blood will be able to maintain an alkaline condition.

As this process continues, these storage areas increase in acidity and some cells die; they then turn themselves into acids. However, some of the cells in this environment may adapt and instead of dying, as normal cells do in an acid environment, some cells survive by becoming abnormal. These are malignant and can grow indefinitely and without order. This is cancer.

Negative ions.

All matter is made up of molecules. These are made up of a dense core of atomic particles including positively charged protons. This core is surrounded by orbiting negatively charged electrons. A normal molecule of air has the same number of protons and electrons making it electrically neutral. However, because an electron is 1,800 times lighter than a proton, the electron is easily displaced. An ion is a molecule that is gained or lost an electron. A negative ion is an air molecule that has gained an electron and a positive ion has lost one. Ions form only a small part of the air we breathe but they're the most important part.

In clean open country air there are usually about 1,000 to 2,000 ions per cubic centimetre but these drop to only a few hundred in a polluted environment or in an enclosed ill-ventilated air-conditioned room.

Negative ions give us the feel-good factor, they stimulate and energise us and they also destroy airborne bacteria and mould spores. But most important of all, they supply a large component of the energy in our blood supply!

Every healthy cell carries a negative charge and brain function, in particular, relies as much on correct electrical signals as it does on chemical transfers. Negative ions help to conduct this vital electric current through the body to ensure optimal cellular functioning.

Negative ion generators are now widely available on the internet. The avalanche circuit at the heart of this invention was thought up by Sir John Cockcroft in the 1960's. It basically mimics the ATP mechanism that is nature's energy producing system!

The mechanism.

A normally functioning immune system is an effective defence against foreign infectious agents and against bodily cells that have become cancerous. The immune regulatory mechanisms are genetically controlled and in humans these genes are located on the short arm of chromosome 6. The main components of the immune system are different forms of blood cells and the complex of chemicals known as the complement cascade. Blood cells originate in the bone marrow, as what are called stem cells, and they become differentiated into different types of blood cells as they pass into the bloodstream.

White blood cells form the most active component of the immune system representing only 1% of the total volume. Red cells also play a role in the body's defence and all blood cells are manufactured in the bone marrow at the rate of 200 million a day.

Red blood cells.

Red blood cells go straight into the circulatory system. As they pass through the lungs they absorb the negatively charged oxygen transporting this through the body and delivering it to the cells. They then absorb the positively charged carbon dioxide released from the cells and let this out through the lungs again. Red blood cells are attracted to carbon dioxide about 200 times more than they're attracted to oxygen and because of this, they're very effective clean up agents in the bloodstream and are an important part of the immune system..

Low frequency current.

The blood circulation system basically provides a low frequency current carrying positively and negatively charged particles to and from all the cells of the body. The cells use this power supply to perform their work.

White blood cells.

There are four main types of white blood cells produced by the bone marrow stem cells, two of these the macrophage and the granulocyte circulate all the time in the bloodstream. These are the prowling predators of the immune system which can recognise and attack foreign or damaged cells. The mechanism they use to do this is electromagnetic!

The regulator.

The other two types of white blood cells are called T-lymphocytes and B-lymphocytes. The Blymphocyte cells distributes themselves around the body and are effective in a complex reaction of all four types of blood cells which is controlled and mediated by the activity of T-lymphocytes. Once T-lymphocyte cells become mature, they migrate to the thymus gland which is part of the regulatory system of the body and is controlled by the mind – by mental states. Because the thymus is controlled by the mind and the emotions, a positive mental attitude to healing is essential. It's the thymus acting in concert with the rest of the glandular system which regulates the immune system response.

The recharge system.

It's the job of red cells to carry oxygen and nutrients around the cells and to clean up the system by carrying waste products and carbon dioxide through the cleansing organs and lungs. During each cycle they pass negatively-charged electrons to the cells which use them and pass back positive charges to be disposed of in the carbon dioxide.

White blood cells circulating in the blood pass through the lungs in the same way as the red cells, but the white cells pick up a very strong negative charge. They absorb negative ions from the air. Negative ions are the core of the immune response since they "charge up" the T-lymphocyte cells which use them in an oxidative burst to kill or counter bacteria, virus or all the array of cellular malfunctions which have a positive charge, including cancer.

Overkill.

In some cases the oxidative burst is 'over the top' and fails to distinguish between the cells it's intended to attack and the normal surrounding tissue. When this arises the immune system is then basically attacking the body and at this point such degenerate illnesses as multiple sclerosis and etc. can set in. This process is reversible.

Summary.

To summarise then, over-acidity in the body caused by a variety of factors, the main one being aberrant diet, is the base cause of cancer. This over-acidity is exacerbated by the air we breathe daily which, apart from being very low in oxygen content these days, is even lower in charged oxygen particles from which our body draws much of its power supply.

Vital life.

It's vital therefore that you understand the need for a good negative ioniser in your bed chamber, your office, your living-room, your meeting rooms and anywhere else where you live for long periods. This is useful in keeping the air's power supply fresh and energetic. Without the input of this ioniser you will be breathing denatured air which your body struggles to thrive on.

ACIDIC WASTE

As you age and eat food which is low in oxygen or has no oxygen in it, you will begin to accumulate acidic waste in your cells.

When your blood supply is under supplied with electrons it will be unable to process this acidic waste which can build up to the point where the cells begin to collapse under acidic stress, then turn into potentially cancerous cells.

Cancer is fundamentally a disease of over-acidification, as are most modern diseases, so buy yourself a good ionizer or several and begin to ingest large quantities of Vitamin C.

Chapter 2

VITAMIN C

As we've seen, arteries carry the negative charges picked up from the oxygen into the body and the veins carry the positive charges in the form of carbon dioxide out of the body. This process follows a three-stage route – air enters the lungs when you breathe in and the oxygen, which has a negative charge, passes this negative charge on to the blood cells in a complex process which involves Vitamin C.

This is how it works.

Vitamin C acts as the bridge allowing oxygen to transfer its negative charge to the blood cells. Vitamin C is the best known and most efficient electron acceptor in nature and acts as a bridge between air and protein (via methylglyoxal) to transfer a charge from the oxygen to the blood cells. Once the blood cell has absorbed the oxygen across the Vitamin C bridge, they distribute this charge throughout the body passing through the walls of the arteries in the form of lymph (which is composed of serum) which bathes every cell in the body with oxygen-rich negative charge that the cells require as a power supply. This power supply supplements and facilitates the workings of its energy production system, adenosine triphosphate.

The mechanism by which the cell absorbs the negatively charged oxygen across the membrane is provided by essential fatty acids. These act as oxygen magnets in the cell membrane drawing it in to do work. So if you don't have the proper functional essential fatty acids at the cellular level, then your cells will not absorb enough oxygen from your bloodstream and you'll be more susceptible to cancer.

Essential fatty acids.

Analysis of a western diet shows a significant preponderance of omega-6 compared to omega-3. Doctors and nutritionists tell us that we are therefore overdosed on omega 6 from our food, whilst being undersupplied with omega-3. This is nonsense. Overdosing on omega-3 can make you more susceptible to illness as shown in the scientific calculation of the optimum omega-6 to 3 ratio published by Cambridge International Institute for Medical Science. This paper points out that fish oil recommendations are worthless or even hazardous to health and that an excess of omega-3 in any form is hazardous.

The key ratio over omega-6 to omega-3 in the body tissues is 4 to 1 and the best sources of these oils are hemp and linseed.

All tissues need essential fatty acids which must come from the diet and for most tissues through the plasma where they're almost entirely transported by lipoproteins, mainly in the cholesterol esters and phospholipids. In a natural environment the consumption of organic and unprocessed EFAs (rather than adulterated oils and trans fats) LDL cholesterol is <u>supposed</u> to be made up of significant amounts of properly functioning parent omega-6. Linoleic acid is not supposed to be harmful. It is the natural transporter of omega-6 and omega-3 into the cells; therefore it's not essential to lower cholesterol but vital to lower the intake of trans fats or processed oils.

The body has no cholesterol sensor in the bloodstream because the absolute number of cholesterol is irrelevant.

The conclusion is that if you are not getting sufficient omega-6 in your diet, then the oxygen will not enter your cells which will suffer hypoxia.

Most cooking oils on the market today are ruined by commercial food processing and these are incorporated into the LDL cholesterol. The consumption and transport of defective, cancer-causing processed oils, causes the LDL cholesterol to act like a 'poison' delivery system. Further yet, it's primarily the adulterated parent omega-6 that clogs the arteries, not saturated fat!

Conclusion.

Accordingly, if insufficient oxygen-rich omega-6 and omega-3 essential fatty acids are transported into the body, then the body's electrically charged bloodstream will not be able to transfer its charge into the cells along with the oxygen and the result will be cellular hypoxia and rapid ageing.

Recommendation (A).

Accordingly, you should cut out commercially prepared (and ruined) cooking oils and processed foods and arm yourself with a clean supply of hemp or linseed oil, a spoonful of which should be taken daily.

WATER.

The human body needs 3 pints of clean, pure water a day to function properly. An adult loses approximately 2.7 pints of water daily as waste excreted through the skin, lungs, kidneys and digestive system. 14% of fluid is made by the body when its working on our behalf and the rest must be taken in daily mostly from drinks (52%) and the remainder 34% from food. A little and often is better as water is able to soak into tissues to help dissolve and excrete waste products.

Dehydration causes insomnia and tiredness, hypertension and headaches, arthritis and heart problems, high cholesterol and dementia. It also contributes significantly to the onset of cancer if it's not available to dissolve the acidic build up.

The best time to drink water is one glass half an hour before taking food – breakfast, lunch and dinner – and a similar amount 2½ hours after each meal. This is the minimum amount of water your body needs i.e. 3 pints each day

Water and ageing.

With increase in age, the water content of the cells of the body decreases, to the point that the ratio of the volume of the body water that is inside the cells to what is outside changes from a figure of 1:1 to almost 0:8. As we age we tend to drink less water and become dehydrated, partly because we lose our thirst sensation progressively from the age of 40 (this correlates with our fall off in bicarbonate which I'll deal with later).

Besides being a solvent, water in the body is a means of transport. It has an essential hydrolytic role in all aspects of the body mechanism – water-dependent chemical reactions. At the cell membrane, the osmotic flow of water can generate a voltage gradient that is stored in the energy pools in the form of ATP and used for cation exchanges, particularly in neuro-transmission. ATP is a chemical source of energy in the body which water helps to manufacture. Water also forms a particular structure pattern and shape that is employed as the adhesive material in the bonds of the cell architecture. There exist small waterways along the length of the nerves that float the packages of material along guidelines called micro tubes. In a dehydrated state, the proteins and enzymes become less efficient and it follows that water regulates all functions of the body.

When there's a shortage of water, some cells will go without a portion of their normal needs and some will get a predetermined ration amount to maintain function. When we lose the thirst sensation and drink less water than the daily requirements, the shutting down of some vascular beds is the only natural alternative to keep blood vessels full.

Water by itself is the best natural diuretic and an adequate diet of water can prevent hypertension, heart failure, bowel cancer, diabetes and a whole range of related illnesses.

We lose our thirst reaction progressively beyond the age of 40 because of the decline in our bicarbonate levels. Other liquids such as tea, coffee and soda are not a substitute for purely natural water that your body needs. It's true that these beverages contain water but they also contain caffeine, alcohol, sugar, salt, bromine and a whole range of chemicals which are dehydrating agents.

The authority on this subject is Dr. F. Batmanghelidj whose book, *"Your Body's Many Cries for Water"*, can be accessed on the internet. If you don't drink sufficient water you increase your susceptibility to a whole range of diseases including cancer.

Recommendation (B).
Drink three pints of water a day spread out through the day and you will help yourself to recover by getting what you need.

Chlorinated water.

Both chlorine and fluoride are halogens which are enzyme disruptive and affect thyroid hormones. As a result, people who drink these substances can develop underactive thyroids which are becoming much more prevalent. These substances also contribute to the appalling rise in clinical obesity because thyroid hormones rely on iodine, which is an element in the same family as chlorine but these can displace iodine in the body leading to problems with the thyroid gland.

How to reduce your exposure to chlorine and fluoride.

1. Avoid having long hot showers and baths unless you've installed a full-house filtration system such as reverse osmosis.

2. Use an activated carbon filter attached to your shower head to reduce levels of chlorine when showering.

3. Swim in salt water or ozone-disinfected swimming pools whenever possible.

4. Filter your tap water before drinking it.

5. Drink bottled water from a good natural source.

6. Use disinfectant bi-product-free water for all drinking and cooking purposes.

7. When dishwashing in unfiltered tap water use rubber gloves.

8. To remove the chlorine from tap water, fill up a jug with tap water and allow it to stand at room temperature for two hours. This will not remove all chlorination bi-products but it's a start.

Chapter 3

IODINE.

Iodine is a vital antioxidant in life's processes. It protects against free radicals (superoxide anion, hydrogen peroxide and hydroxyl radical that oxygen breeds). Iodine increases the antioxidant status of human serum similar to but on a different vector from Vitamin C.

Iodine induces programmed cell death. This process is essential to growth and development and is also vital for destroying cells that represent a threat to the integrity of the organism (like cancer cells).

Russian researchers first showed in 1966 that iodine effectively relieves signs and symptoms of fibrocystic breast disease and in 1993 a Canadian study published in the Canadian Journal of Surgery, likewise found that iodine relieves signs and symptoms of fibrocystic breast disease in 70% of their patients.

The FDA regard iodine as a natural substance not a drug and most physicians and surgeons view iodine from a narrow perspective as an antiseptic that disinfects drinking water and prevents surgical wounds' infection. It's also needed by the thyroid to make thyroid hormones.

The thyroid gland needs iodine to synthesise hormones that regulate metabolism and steer growth and development and whilst the thyroid only needs trace elements of iodine, there's a vast body of evidence that a higher dose of iodine will prevent a whole spectrum of disorders. The Nobel Laureate Dr. Albert Szent-Györgyi (1893 to 1986), the physician who discovered Vitamin C, widely recommended iodine's use as a sort of universal medicine.

To maintain whole body sufficiency of iodine requires 12.5 milligram a day. This is similar to what the Japanese consume with the seaweed in their diet. The vast majority of people retain a substantial amount of this dosage and many require 50 milligrams a day for several months before they excrete 90% of it, indicating that their body has reached its equilibrium. In fact the body will hold 1,500 milligram with only 3% of that being held in the thyroid gland. Thyroid function remains unchanged using this amount of iodine and since it removes toxic halogens, fluoride and bromide from the body, we should all take at least 2 drops of Lugol's solution or 1 iodoral tablet a day.

Until recently the chief source of iodine in the western diet was table salt. However, the bulk of people now buy salt without iodine which is called table salt but has all the trace elements driven off. Accordingly, over the last three decades people who used to use iodised table salt have now unwittingly decreased their consumption by 65%. Moreover, high concentrations of chloride in manufactured salt inhibit absorption of its sister halogen iodine.

The intestines only absorb 10% of the iodine present in iodised table salt, so in order to stay healthy it's vital to increase one's intake of iodine. You will find that everything in your body functions better (even your brain) once it's nourished by the iodine it needs. The key here is to think of iodine not as a remedy but as a nutrient that's crucial to all aspects of health and can help enormously in recovery from cancer.

Your doctor will probably say that you get all the iodine you need from fish and if you could consume 20 lbs of fish a day and withstand the mercury, PCPs and etc. now present in all fish you probably could! However, 2 drops of Lugol's per day in a glass of water is safe and an extremely conservative dose and you might like to take more to help yourself recover.

Iodine supplement brings about an immediate lifting of spirits in mildly depressed people and does wonders to alleviate crankiness. It also helps banish long-established migraines!

Finally, because iodine in the cells prevents the uptake of radioactive iodine (a different substance) then iodine is extremely effective in preventing you from suffering from mild radiation poisoning which we're all susceptible to with the increase in background radiation caused by atomic testing and atomic reactor disasters.

Our current exposure to toxicalytes, fluoride, bromide, tetrachlorates and isocyanate is higher than humans have ever been exposed to in the past. Fluoride, a strong neuro-toxin, is added to drinking water, allegedly to stop tooth decay, and we also ingest fluoride from sources such as pesticides, medicines, food, salt, toothpaste and health supplements.

Similarly, bromide is another toxic halide which is everywhere. It's got an antibacterial function similar to chlorine and is used as a fumigant for agriculture and termites. It's a virulent pesticide that kills insects on contact and when it's injected into the soil everything dies.

It's cheap and abundant and appears in a vast number of food stuffs and has replaced iodine as a dough conditioner for bread and is used widely in the milk industry because of its effective bactericide properties.

This is where iodine comes in. It helps the body eliminate fluoride, bromide, lead, calcium, arsenic, aluminium and mercury, and since it's now been replaced by bromine in bread and milk, there's no longer a way to eliminate the bromine.

The ubiquitous nature of bromide in food stuffs, particularly sodas, gives rise to morbid obesity. When oil is placed in a bowl and bromine is stirred in, the bromine will slowly turn the liquid oil into a solid until it becomes so stiff that the spoon won't move. This happens in your body and goes a long way toward explaining the cause of our epidemic of obesity. Years of drinking sodas that are loaded with brominated vegetable oil solidifies body fat.

To conclude, adequate iodine levels are necessary for proper immune system function. About 1.5 billion people around the world live in areas of iodine deficiency and iodine is responsible for the production of all the hormones of the body and 20% of the body store of iodine is in the skin.

Accordingly, if you want to recover your health as quickly as possible, it is vital that you begin to use iodine as part of your diet.

MORE ON VITAMIN C, VITAMIN E AND SELENIUM

We all suffer from hypo-ascorbaemia, a deficiency of ascorbate in the blood, or in other words a lack of Vitamin C. Human beings with a high intake of Vitamin C manufacture more antibody molecules than those with a lower intake. Antibodies or antitoxins are protein molecules which have the power of recognising "not self" cells and combining with them thus helping to mark them for destruction by the body's normal processes.

Self and not self

There is another complex of protein molecules called complement that is involved in an essential way in the process of destruction of foreign and malignant cells. It's been shown that an increased intake of Vitamin C significantly increases the amount of the first component of complement, C1 esterase, without which the whole complement cascade is inoperable.

Scurvy

Pioneering research into the relationship between Vitamin C deficiency and heart disease began in the late 1940s not long after the structure of Vitamin C was determined. Canadian doctors proved that a Vitamin C deficiency causes the condition commonly called scurvy. These doctors found that the condition will arise in 100% of Vitamin C deprived animals tested and in subjects that don't make their own Vitamin C (like for instance humans).

Vitamin C has many actions in the body and an important one being its antioxidant activity. This inhibits cancer reliably with experimental animals and it also confers resistance to the progress of cancer, even after it's established in the body.

Patients supplemented with Vitamin C have a death rate from cancer between 40 and 60% less than those on normal diets. This decrease in death rate gives an increased life span of 8 to 11 years. Dr Linus Pauling, the two-time Nobel Laureate, finally convinced the National Cancer Institute of the vitamin's benefits, but this has yet to be widely recognised and used by the medical profession.

Vitamin E

Another vitamin which has known effects on cancer is Vitamin E. It's very important because of its antioxidant activity, especially in the protection of cell membranes. Along with Vitamin C and selenium, it's also important in protecting the intestines and colon as some of it fails to be digested and passes through the body with food wastes. Vitamin E is fat-soluble, it retards putrefaction of faecal fat and colon walls are therefore subjected to less potential injury.

SELENIUM

The mineral selenium is essential for the immune system and has a number of potentially anti-cancer actions. An editorial in the British Medical Journal points to the fact that the UKRDA is 70mcg/day and suggests that the rise in cancer might well be due to wide-spread selenium depletion. A further recent study in London indicates that selenium can force cancer cells to commit suicide at 200mcg and since selenium is essential for C43, the membrane proteins involved in cell contact inhibition and switching off cell growth, then selenium is highly recommended as an essential mineral addition to the vitamin recommendations laid out here.

The fact that the human organism evolved to eat large quantities of Vitamin C and Vitamin E daily is indicated because part of the natural function of these nutrients in the human body is to pass through it along with food residues to directly protect the bowels and bladder from injurious effects of the body's own waste during the process of their elimination.

In 1977 the eminent British cancer specialist, Sir Richard Doll, echoed the feelings of many nutritionists when he said, *"I've laid particular stress on diet because I suspect in the next few years the main advance in our knowledge of how to control cancer will come from studying this aspect in our environment"*. In the distant past when we lived on a normal healthy diet, we simply didn't get cancer because the diet prevented it. Therefore the cause of cancer is modern lifestyle and its cure is only to be achieved through correct nutrition.

More on Scurvy

Dr. Irwin Stone published a paper in the 1980s entitled *"Scurvy, the most misunderstood epidemic disease in the 20th century"*. This paper has considerable implications for cancer patients because the poor and inadequate correction of the human defective gene for GLO (too little ascorbate daily intake) causes every cancer victim to be born scorbutic, after a nine month intra-uterine bout with scurvy.

This poor correlation due to grossly inadequate intakes of ascorbate continues through the lifetime of the victims exposing them constantly to the deleterious physiological insults of chronic, subclinical scurvy which is a large factor in the genesis of cancer.

How much?

Every individual is different and the amount will depend on personal physiology. Everyone has an ideal dose that will be discovered through an element of trial and error. By taking a series of incremental doses every four hours your body will reach a tolerance level known as the bowel tolerance threshold. This is the state where the tissue cells have become fully saturated with the maximum amount needed for the body to heal itself. Bowel tolerance threshold is not diarrhoea as it's not acidic and will not create the burning sensation associated with diarrhoea. At the bowel tolerance threshold the dose can be reduced by small amounts to come below the threshold. By a process of trial and error I now take between 8 and 10 grams a day which, at age 75, I find to be adequate to keep me in good condition.

Incidentally, the regime every four hours does not need to be continued during the night, but simply begun again in the morning. This regime can be followed preventatively for long-term tissue and organ healing and it helps wonderfully against cancer.

Finally, there are two types of ascorbic acid on the market, straightforward ascorbic acid and sodium ascorbate. It's a myth that sodium will raise blood pressure, but for a very small minority of people who are truly hyper sensitive, sodium MAY raise blood pressure levels, this being dependent on many factors including the ratio of potassium. In such cases ascorbic acid can be taken instead of the salt of ascorbic acid and it should be noted that sodium ascorbate contains only 10% of sodium (unlikely to do you any harm – quite the reverse).

Bioflavonoids

Taking ascorbic acid – Vitamin C by itself is not a good idea. You need to take it with the additional bioflavonoids and rosehip extract. These catalyse its activity and mimic the way that it's presented to you in nature. So look for a source of 1,000 milligram Vitamin C tablets that contain citrus bioflavonoids and rosehips.

Chapter 4

CHARCOAL.

Everything alive on earth today is, as far as we know, carbon based. Until recently it was thought there were only three basic types of carbon available on earth and none of those were capable of providing a structure on which life could evolve. Graphite is too malleable – diamond is too rigid and far too hard and soot is formless. So the type of carbon upon which life was based was until recently a mystery. However, in 1985 carbon C_{60} was discovered and this is now called fullerene after Buckminster Fuller, the famous architect. (C_{60} has a geodesic structure like the geodesic dome invented by Buckminster Fuller.)

C_{60} is hollow like a ball and only three angstroms across, just enough space to enclose one other atom in its structure. So C_{60} which is pure carbon has a form of structure which is strong, resilient and biologically active. It can combine with other elements.

Adsorption

C_{60} activate or potentised charcoal has a unique ability to adsorb toxins. This adsorption process causes atoms or molecules of a substance to form on or bind to its surface. Tiny particles of charcoal are riddled with a network of crevices, cracks and tunnels such that the combined surface area of a one centimetre cube would unfold to a 1,000 square centimetres. This tremendous surface area is capable of adsorbing well over 4,000 acidic substances by physically binding molecules to the charcoal in a process known as van der Waal forces.

Van der Waal forces are electromagnetic in nature and there is a vast body of scientific evidence showing that C_{60} charcoal not only adsorbs over 4,000 different toxic substances, but also carries (owing to its electron cloud) a substantial burst of energy into the body where it is used to capture and transmit free radicals (excess electrons left over from an oxidative burst) guiding these down the metabolic pathways of the body.

Charcoal derived carbon C_{60} is used by the body to build a healthy carbon network which forms all important pathways along which oxygen moves. In its absence, oxygen burned in the cells as fuel forms free radicals which are an oxygen species which can do great harm, but when oxygen is "burned" by the cells in the presence of $C_{60,}$ this forms a spherical cage around the rogue oxygen species and reinstalls them in their proper respiratory pathways. Effectively this activity acts also as an antiviral, antifungal and antibacterial mechanism. It doesn't kill these three, but simply deactivates them by temporarily neutralising their positively charged nucleic acids - i.e. they are less of a threat whilst in the presence of C_{60}-rich charcoal molecules.

Finally, C_{60} charcoal has an affinity for acidic toxins adsorbing over 4,000 known elements of these species. By adsorbing acidic toxins from the gut and bloodstream and indeed from the entire system, this helps to rebalance the pH in the body helping it to become more alkaline, and therefore better oxygenated. In this role charcoal C_{60} performs a vital function in the recovery of cells' energy levels helping to switch them back from cancer (the dark state of life) into normal healthy cells driven by the citrate cycle – light life.

The C_{60} molecule prevents free radical damage by forming a spherical cage around them (i.e. the free radicals) and reinstalling them in their proper respiratory pathways. It also revitalises the health of cells which are "run down" and losing their shape. This is a vital function in that it restores their ability to carry oxygen! Ergo, it provides a reliable and stable template for cellular rheology. This is a critical step in the process of reviving cancerous cells and turning them back into normal body cells.

If you take 2 - 4 x 250mg charcoal capsules every night with a glass of water, not only will your entire system become a lot more healthy, courtesy of the detox, but the energy that this wonderful substance transmits throughout the body will help your cells recover their true identity.

Chapter 5

TURMERIC

The highly sophisticated ancient medicine system of India which dates back over 6,000 years is called Ayurveda. This has turmeric as a remedy for many ills. Turmeric, which is the dried rhizome of curcuma longa, has been used for centuries as a spice, food preservative and colouring agent which has been found to be a rich source of phenolic compounds collectively termed curcuminoids. Although the chemical structure was determined in 1910, it was only around the early 1980s that the potential uses of curcuminoid compounds in medicine began to be extensively studied in the West. The potential use in the prevention of cancer has been now well established and the antioxidant properties of curcuminoids well established.

The trade-off

Oxygen is crucial for the metabolism, functioning and well-being of the body. However, metabolism comes with certain costs which are known as oxygen bi-products. They become wastes that pollute the body and causes damage to DNA (genetic material which is a blueprint for the cells' organisational centre) and inflammation.

Inflammation is encountered in the course of certain diseases, for example, arthritis, infection or wound healing and is nothing more than the outcome of the defence reaction of the body producing oxidants that cause collateral damage to tissue and organs. Moderate inflammation is necessary for the healing process, whereas continuous inflammation leads to chronic conditions like arthritis and associated pain.

The role of antioxidants is a complex one and many antioxidants recycle other antioxidant nutrients that have been oxidised or spent in sacrifice to free radicals. Individual antioxidants' nutrients differ in their transport and storage, some acting primarily in the aqueous portion of the bloodstream, others within particles of lipoprotein in the blood, others on cell membranes and still others within cellular cytoplasm (and even a few in cell nuclei). The antioxidant profile of Vitamin E is different from that of Vitamin C and the antioxidant properties of curcuminoids (turmeric) are different once again.

Turmeric works to protect the genetic material within the cell and damp down free radical activity preventing the transmission of radical molecules from surrounding cells. Since disorganised cell growth usually results in cancer, the need for antioxidants like turmeric to stop free radical damage is well recognised. Curcuminoids act as bio-protectants, being natural plant compounds that guard the cells, tissues and organs of the body from numerous inside and outside influences.

Basically, the curcuminoids are able to absorb many of the negative characteristics of free radicals, thus preventing their formation. As a comparison with fat soluble Vitamin E, curcumin is eight times more powerful in preventing lipid peroxidation.

Anticancer activity

The nutritional role of turmeric extract and curcuminoids, as anti-carcinogens in preventing the development of cancer and as anti-mutagens in preventing damage to genetic material, has been widely researched.

Curcuminoids exhibit antimicrobial properties inhibiting the growth of numerous gram-positive and gram-negative bacteria, fungi and internal parasites. Since cancerous cells display many aspects of fungi, turmeric and its active principles the curcuminoids, can exert protection by shielding the biomolecular functioning of the body and by boosting the immune system function.

Fundamentally, turmeric extract and curcuminoids act as antifungal agents which, since cancer is a fungal type outgrowth, can prove enormously effective in protecting you.

Chapter 6

ALKALINITY/ACIDITY

Scientists unanimously agree that free-radical activity is the basis of chronic disease such as cancer and the ageing process. One of the best ways to combat this damaging process is to supply the body with more oxygen which is the penultimate store of electrons. By supplying more oxygen, we're supplying the body with the means to shut down the excess immune response by providing the free radicals the means to regain their stable state. This doesn't reduce the immune system but enables it to distinguish better between damaged tissue and healthy tissue and therefore do its job better.

pH

A healthy body functions properly when it's slightly alkaline. Deviations in the blood above or below a pH range of 7.30 to 7.45 signals potentially dangerous symptoms or states of disease. When your solent tissues' pH levels deviate from a healthy range (7.2 to 7.5) to an acidic state (below 7.0 pH) the acid waste normally discarded through the body's elimination routes starts to back up and clog the system.

SODIUM BICARBONATE

To counter this, the human body produces a balancing factor of high alkalinity which is bicarbonate (HCO_3). Bicarbonate keeps the blood alkaline and various stomach lining glands produce mucous that has a pH of 7.7 and contains large quantities (up to .5 grams a day) of sodium bicarbonate. This alkaline mucous protects the stomach from its own acid and under normal conditions, for each molecule of acid produced, one of sodium bicarbonate is also produced.

Alkaline tide

Blood leaving the stomach is relatively alkaline that is rich in bicarbonate and short of chloride. As this alkaline tide circulates around the body, its raised alkalinity helps to reduce any acidosis that has built up. So bicarbonate keeps the blood alkaline.

In 1996 Dr. Lynda Frassetto of the University of California, San Francisco, published a paper showing how bicarbonate levels in human blood vary with age.

The average bicarbonate level is constant until the age of 45, after which it noticeably begins to decline. It is the age when symptoms of diabetes, arthritis, hypertension, osteoporosis and cancer start to appear. As the bicarbonate level declines, the acidity of the bloodstream rises and it's this major swing in the acidity of our diet that has dramatically shortened life. To bring our systems back into balance we need to ingest potassium which is plentiful in vegetables and fruits and produces strong alkalizing ions in body fluids.

The attached food list gives an indication of the pH rating of a great many foods from which you should choose those with an alkaline rating.

Cooking

For millions of years we lived on raw food. Raw or living food is full of enzymes, vitamins and minerals. It really feeds the body and most people report that they instantly feel better following a raw food diet. There are roughly 80 million species on earth, about 700,000 of which are animals, and all of these species thrive on raw food. Only humans apply heat to what they eat and on average as a race, die at or below half their potential life span.

Microscopic burnt nutrients (resulting from heated food) are toxic to the body and as decades pass by, the harmful effects of consuming these toxins accumulate. Cooking denatures protein, altering it, making it either unusable or less useable. Heated proteins are unavailable to the body and coagulated protein molecules tend to putrefy as bacteria and feed on dead organic matter.

Protein consumed is not used as protein, but first broken down into its individual amino acids and then used to build the protein molecules that the body needs. So, animal flesh products must be broken down, using up energy. Raw food has an abundance of readily available amino acids, especially ripe fruit, vegetables, nuts and seeds. Accordingly, the body has a lot less work to do when creating protein from the assortment of individual amino acids from greens.

Scientific research proves that raw food protects against cancer and decreases toxic products in the colon. A raw, vegan diet causes a reduction in the bacterial enzymes and toxic products that have been implicated in colon cancer. The risk of breast cancer is also lower.

Vitamins and minerals

Up to 50% of vitamins and minerals are destroyed by heat. Minerals are altered and become less absorbable. 100% of enzymes are damaged which depletes the body's supply draining the energy needed to maintain and repair tissue and organ systems. Depleted food devoid of enzymes as a result of cooking, food irradiation and microwaving causes an enlargement of the pancreas and causes stress to associated endocrine glands such as the adrenals, pituitary, ovaries and testes. The human pancreas is three times larger compared to total body weight and that of any other animal and is thought that the pancreas becomes enlarged because it's forced to keep up a high digestive enzyme output!

It's no coincidence that since 1950, as consumption of processed foods has increased, so have cancer rates.

You can still enjoy cooked foods and be healthy to some degree by food combining. This allows the digestion to operate smoothly without food fermenting and putrefying in your digestive system. However, to aim for the ideal diet with which we evolved, 83% of your diet should be raw food.

Sodium bicarbonate supplementation

We've seen that sodium bicarbonate levels begin to decline around 40 which is usually around the time when the major dread diseases begin to manifest. In 2005, Dr. Tullio Simoncini, an eminent Italian oncologist, published a theory that cancer is in fact a common fungus, candida. He developed a therapy based upon the use of sodium bicarbonate as a strongly alkaline antifungal. With this theory he practiced his skills on a variety of cancer patients with a <u>90% success rate.</u>

It's worth noting here that the general remission rate of cancer in the wider world is about 7% and the overall 'cure' rate, when treated with standard oncological methodology, is next to nil over time.

This argues significantly that cancer is indeed a fungus and when you look at nature, you see that the true role of fungus is the breakdown of defunct living structures in order to make their component nutrients available again.

Incidentally, Dr. Simoncini should be given the Nobel Prize for this work, since not only is he an outstanding humanitarian, but a profoundly intelligent and perceptive doctor. I suggest you begin to alkalize your system now by drinking a pint of water a day with half a teaspoonful of sodium bicarbonate dissolved in it.

At the end of this book I outline a complete regime by which you can help yourself, so please read on.

Chapter 7

FASTING – RESTRICTED DIET

We are structured to be a hungry hominid. According to the structures of our palate and our gut, we have evolved to live on masses of raw fruit, shoots, nuts and vegetation with very occasional (and often dangerous) intakes of raw meat. We are designed with digestive systems capable of getting the very maximum energy and food value out of a wide range of diets and we are evolved to live very well on very little food. Until about 10,000 years ago we lived as hunter-gatherers and the rhythms of such life meant enduring long and regular periods of hunger. We're actually structured to respond to wide fluctuations in food supply and to go hungry or slightly hungry for much of the time.

Unless you're doing hard physical work, you do not need to take in large amounts of food each day. On the contrary, you need to take in, to eat, small amounts of the right food regularly.

Raw vegetation or fibrous matter is often quite high in cellulose which is difficult for our digestive systems to break down and use. To facilitate the use of this food, which in our recent past formed our main diet, we evolved a sacculated bowel. This structure slows down the rate at which our food is evacuated and allows the movement of the body to massage the lower abdomen so as to work or knead partially digested food as it passes through the intestines. (This is why walking after a meal can help digestion.) The sacculations in the bowel evolved to aid in the digestion of simple vegetable and fruit material rich in its own enzymes and it has just the opposite effect on meat. They slow it down dangerously.

All carnivores have smooth bowels. These enable them to eat fresh killed meat, full of the fear hormone adrenalin and very poorly supplied with natural enzymes. Their systems can take what they need very quickly from this rapidly decaying toxin mass and then get rid of the residues very quickly through their bowels so as to avoid the bulk of toxic absorption.

Untreated toxins derived from unnatural food in the bowel flood the body. This is the root cause of most illnesses.

Throughout history, both religion and philosophy have laid great emphasis on regular fasting as a method of clearing the mind and purifying the body.

If we stop eating for a time, our body's work away steadily and use up all the food matter available in our intestines. Everything is gradually broken down and used and this process continues until nothing is left.

Then, and only then, does the body begin to use its reserves of stored fat and as these are processed into glucose, the toxins they often contain are dealt with by the immune system often being excreted through the skin as perspiration.

Finally, the bloodstream is cleaned of all toxins and foreign matter by the enzymes and white blood corpuscles and the body becomes completely healthy.

At this point the bowel becomes completely sterile!

Under 45 years of age, if kept short of food, your body will usually revert to a more alkaline state. In this condition it will often metabolize tumors as food and they will disappear. This may be why fat people may get cancer more often than slim people.

After 45, as the bicarb element declines, this process is unlikely to take place or will take place much less quickly and can be accelerated, as I said before, by adding small quantities of bicarbonate dissolved in water into your diet.

With knowledge of the foregoing, it's obvious that the human body is perfectly capable of clearing up almost any illness, left to its own devices to do so.

Begin to fast one day a week and you will notice a very rapid improvement in your health. If you find this impossible to do, then simply halve the quantity of food that you take in at each meal and stop eating yourself into an early grave.

Chapter 8

BLOOD CLEANSE

As your body begins to right itself using the methods that I have listed in this book, your immune system can begin to destroy cancerous cells and ultimately tumors.

These break down into fungal-type microbes and toxins which can be very damaging if left to accumulate in the bloodstream. In severe cases they can lead to massive inflammations and infections which sometimes result in death from lung infections or liver failure. In other extreme cases people die from cachexia which is severe weight loss and muscle wasting due to progressive anemia caused by the destruction of red blood cells by fungal microbes.

In order to avoid this unhappy ending, it is vital that anyone using the regime that I have outlined above, use natural proteolytic enzymes which help to remove protein debris and shrink tumors at the same time as powering down inflammation. Amongst these, papain and bromelain are amongst the most effective and the fibrinolytic enzymes serrapeptase and nattokinase are useful to help prevent excessive blood clumping or the hyper coagulation needed for metastasis to form.

Similarly, an anti-parasitic regime is strongly recommended with three herbs being used together. Black walnut hull and wormwood kill adults and development stages of at least 100 parasites. Cloves kill the eggs. If you use them together, you'll rid yourself of parasites, which have built up in the acidic environment of your body, which in turn will remove many of the acidic poisons now swishing round your system.

A word of caution, black walnut hulls, wormwood and common cloves should be taken together, not separately, and these will help clean up your system wonderfully and hasten your recovery.

CONCLUSION

By enriching the air you breathe with a **negative ionizer**, which in turn will provide your bloodstream with an abundant supply of electrons which enter the bloodstream and are transferred by Vitamin C to the blood cells, you're beginning the recharge process. By consuming **essential fatty acids** from linseed and hemp, your body's electrically charged bloodstream will transfer its charge into the cells, along with the oxygen and by taking sufficient **water**, you'll provide a means of transport which helps to generate a voltage gradient across the cell membrane, thus helping the adenosine triphosphate to generate more energy. By using **iodine** you help your thyroid gland to synthesize hormones that regulate metabolism and steer growth (which prevent a whole spectrum of disorders). The iodine will also help considerably to eliminate the modern poisons, fluoride, bromide, lead, calcium, arsenic, aluminum and mercury. This takes the weight off your immune system and by taking large doses of **Vitamin C**,

Vitamin E and **selenium**, you are not only boosting your electromagnetic function, but also protecting yourself from the injurious effects of ingested poisons from your diet and the body's own waste. (You're also considerably reducing incidents of scurvy, from which most of us suffer.)

Then by taking **charcoal C_{60}**, you are cleaning up the acidic toxins which have accumulated in your digestive system, whilst at the same time rebuilding your healthy carbon network which forms all important pathways along which oxygen moves. Because C_{60} donates a substantial level of electrons to the cells, you are then going further to increase cellular-energy levels and by taking **turmeric**, you are going some way toward completing a full-spectrum antioxidant rescue. I say full spectrum because turmeric, Vitamin C, Vitamin E, and selenium, whilst working in conjunction with each other, each work in a different way to both absorb many of the negative characteristics of free radicals and preventing their formation in the first place.

The carbon C_{60} molecule donates a more energy-rich load via the white blood corpuscles, throughout the body. This is a gradual process which takes time but which is significantly assisted by a change of diet to incorporate a substantial degree of raw food in your diet.

You should also pay attention to the attached food list and concentrate on increasing the number of **alkaline foods** in your diet so as to give yourself the best possible chance to thoroughly alkalize your system when it may well be able to overcome cancer.

Then by switching to a predominantly **raw food diet** cutting out processed foods and reducing the amount of cooked food that you eat, you will dramatically increase your store of enzymes which help with your digestion and also begin to increase the alkalinity of your system. At this point half a teaspoonful of **sodium bicarbonate** taken with your now numerous glasses of water throughout the day will progressively shrink tumors gradually without causing inflammation, since bicarbonate alkalizes the lymph and inhibits inflammation so that, as long as the alkalinity is maintained, the shrinking tumors don't cause a problem, since bicarbonate inhibits the inflammation that would otherwise occur through too rapid a treatment.

FASTING

Finally, we turn to fasting. This is perhaps the hardest part of the whole regime since our species is programmed to eat when food is available and we rarely get enough exercise.

To begin fasting, cut out all sugars from your diet. Sugar is an addictive toxin-forming-highly-acidic substance (only found in tiny quantities in nature) and one which is almost completely foreign to our systems.

If you can cut out sugar for two or three weeks, then you'll find your taste perceptions change and it becomes much easier to fast.

Fast one day a week and only drink water on that day (with the added bicarb I've recommended) and you will gradually find it easier to fast for longer periods.

If you really can't bring yourself or discipline yourself to fasting, then cut down your intake of food by half. Spare eating which gives your body time to digest your food properly has long been recognized as the secret to overall good health.

FINAL THOUGHTS

At the beginning of this book I mentioned that cancer is a fungus or has fungal-like characteristics in the body. I suspect that the similarity to fungi such as candida albicans which is present throughout the body, is simply nature's way of adapting and using a familiar pattern to achieve a similar end.

Since that end is the breakdown of increasingly unviable living matter, then it's really a moot point as to what it is as long as it responds to treatment.

Accordingly, there is a great deal of epidemiological evidence to the effect that cancer responds to antifungal treatment.

One of the best known antifungal treatments is an increase in temperature. Fungus is temperature sensitive and if you can maintain a high body temperature, you will help to rid yourself of cancer. Similarly, a reduction in carbohydrate intake will help, because we are still structured by our evolution to live on a Paleolithic-type diet rich in nuts, vegetables, lean meats and not much in the way of carbohydrates.

Apricot kernels which contain a high proportion of the vitamin laetrile vitamin B17 are a well-known route to putting cancer into remission and even such extreme sounding remedies as turpentine and benzoic acid have in the past played a significant role in putting cancer into remission.

Simply put, it's now widely accepted that cancer is a fungal form and if you treat it with non-poisonous fungicides, over a period of time it should go into remission!

MY DAILY DOSAGES

1. I take between 8 and 10 grams (1,000 milligram tablets) of Vitamin C as ascorbic acid with citrus bioflavonoids and rosehips which come in the same tablet. (This is my maintenance dose).
2. I also take 400 milligram of turmeric twice a day
3. Two 1000 milligram linseed vegetable pods
4. 400 international units of Vitamin E mixed tocopherols
5. 50 pica-grams of selenium
6. One Vitamin B complex tablet
7. One 5,000 international unit capsule of Vitamin D3 and Vitamin K2 combined,
8. 150 milligram of magnesium,
9. 15 milligram of zinc with copper
10. Two drops of Lugol's iodine daily in a small glass of water before breakfast
11. I also take one high-quality vegetable sourced multivitamin each day
12. 120 milligram coenzyme Q10 capsule.

13. 5 x 250mg capsules of potentised charcoal C_{60} capsules last thing at night with water.
14. I work with negative ionizers beside my bed, on my desk and in my sitting-room.
15. I walk barefoot at least a mile a day through the countryside so as to absorb the maximum air energy available and I maintain a positive attitude through the practice of meditation and yoga.
16. I take ½ a teaspoon of sodium bicarbonate dissolved in a pint of water every morning first thing, before a cup of lemon tea. This gets me off to a good start every day and helps keep my system slightly alkaline.

NOTE: These are spread throughout the day so as not to over-alkalize my system at any one time.

Also, I have a complete break from all of the above for a few days every month to give my system a 'rest'.

CACHEXIA.

Cachexia describes severe weight loss and muscle wasting due to progressive anemia from the destruction of red blood cells by fungal-type blood microbes. These occur in abundance in cancerous conditions and by surrounding the blood cells are effectively able to prevent them from carrying oxygen round the body. Basically, these cancer causing microbes block the oxidity of energy production of affected cells when they start producing energy anaerobically as I've described earlier. The problem we face then in altering the acid-alkaline balance in the body is that if we alkalize the system too quickly, then the cancerous condition "defends itself" with a release of substantial amounts of toxins which cause chronic inflammation. This inflammation, as we've seen, can cause a serious overreaction on the part of the immune system.

Therefore, proceed slowly to give your body time to adjust and gradually re-oxygenate your entire system.

The Answer to Cancer – An Electron Deficit Condition

PART 2

Chapter 9

pH Foods List

The pH scale runs from pH 0 for very strong acid (e.g. battery acid) to pH 14 for very strong alkali (e.g. liquid drain cleaner) a pH of 7 being neutral (e.g. "pure" water).

Alkaline Forming Foods

VEGETABLES	FRUITS	OTHER
Garlic	Apple	Apple Cider Vinegar
Asparagus	Apricot	Bee Pollen
Fermented Veggies	Avocado	Lecithin Granules
Watercress	Banana (high	Probiotic Cultures
Beets	glycemic)	Green Juices
Broccoli	Cantaloupe	Veggies Juices
Brussel sprouts	Cherries	Fresh Fruit Juice
Cabbage	Currants	Organic Milk
Carrot	Dates/Figs	(unpasteurized)
Cauliflower	Grapes	Mineral Water
Celery	Grapefruit	Alkaline Antioxidant
Chard	Lime	Water
Chlorella	Honeydew Melon	Green Tea
Collard Greens	Nectarine	Herbal Tea
Cucumber	Orange	Dandelion Tea
Eggplant	Lemon	Ginseng Tea
Kale	Peach	Banchi Tea
Kohlrabi	Pear	Kombucha
Lettuce	Pineapple	
Mushrooms	All Berries	**SWEETENERS**
Mustard Greens	Tangerine	Stevia
Dulse	Tomato	Ki Sweet
Dandelions	Tropical Fruits	
Edible Flowers	Watermelon	**SPICES/SEASONINGS**
Onions		Cinnamon
Parsnips (high	**PROTEIN**	Curry
glycemic)	Eggs (poached)	Ginger

The Answer to Cancer – An Electron Deficit Condition

Peas	Whey Protein	Mustard
Peppers	Powder	Chili Pepper
Pumpkin	Cottage Cheese	Sea Salt
Rutabaga	Chicken Breast	Miso
Sea Vegetables	Yogurt	Tamari
Spirulina	Almonds	All Herbs
Sprouts	Chestnuts	
Squashes	Tofu (fermented)	**ORIENTAL**
Alfalfa	Flax Seeds	**VEGETABLES**
Barley Grass	Pumpkin Seeds	Maitake
Wheat Grass	Tempeh	Daikon
Wild Greens	(fermented)	Dandelion Root
Nightshade Veggies	Squash Seeds	Shitake
	Sunflower Seeds	Kombu
	Millet	Reishi
	Sprouted Seeds	Nori
	Nuts	Umeboshi
		Wakame
		Sea Veggies

Acid Forming Foods

FATS & OILS	**NUTS & BUTTERS**	**DRUGS &**
Avocado Oil	Cashews	**CHEMICALS**
Canola Oil	Brazil Nuts	Aspartame
Corn Oil	Peanuts	Chemicals
Hemp Seed Oil	Peanut Butter	Drugs, Medicinal
Flax Oil	Pecans	Drugs, Psychedelic
Lard	Tahini	Pesticides
Olive Oil	Walnuts	Herbicides
Safflower Oil		
Sesame Oil	**ANIMAL PROTEIN**	**ALCOHOL**
Sunflower Oil	Beef	Beer
	Carp	Spirits
FRUITS	Clams	Hard Liquor
Cranberries	Fish	Wine
	Lamb	
GRAINS	Lobster	**BEANS & LEGUMES**
Rice Cakes	Mussels	Black Beans
Wheat Cakes	Oyster	Chick Peas
Amaranth	Pork	Green Peas

The Answer to Cancer – An Electron Deficit Condition

Barley Buckwheat Corn Oats (rolled) Quinoa Rice (all) Rye Spelt Kamut Wheat Hemp Seed Flour **DAIRY** Cheese, Cow Cheese, Goat Cheese, Processed Cheese, Sheep Milk Butter	Rabbit Salmon Shrimp Scallops Tuna Turkey Venison **PASTA (WHITE)** Noodles Macaroni Spaghetti **OTHER** Distilled Vinegar Wheat Germ Potatoes	Kidney Beans Lentils Lima Beans Pinto Beans Red Beans Soy Beans Soy Milk White Beans Rice Milk Almond Milk

Extremely Alkaline Forming Foods - pH 8.5 to 9.0	Extremely Acid Forming Foods - pH 5.0 to 5.5
9.0 Lemons, Watermelon	**5.0** Artificial sweeteners
8.5 Agar Agar, Cantaloupe, Cayenne (Capsicum), Dried dates & figs, Kelp, Karengo, Kudzu root, Limes, Mango, Melons, Papaya, Parsley, Seedless grapes (sweet), Watercress, Seaweeds, Asparagus, Endive, Kiwifruit, Fruit juices, Grapes (sweet), Passion fruit, Pears (sweet), Pineapple, Raisins, Umeboshi plum, Vegetable juices	**5.5** Beef, Carbonated soft drinks & fizzy drinks, Cigarettes (tailor made), Drugs, Flour (white, wheat) Goat, Lamb, Pastries & cakes from white flour, Pork, Sugar (white) Beer, Brown sugar, Chicken, Deer, Chocolate, Coffee, Custard with white sugar, Jams, Jellies, Liquor, Pasta (white), Rabbit, Semolina, Table salt refined and iodized, Tea black, Turkey, Wheat bread, White rice, White vinegar (processed).

The Answer to Cancer – An Electron Deficit Condition

Moderate Alkaline – ph 7.5 to 8.0	Moderate Acid - pH 6.0 to 6.5
8.0 Apples (sweet), Apricots, Alfalfa sprouts, Arrowroot Flour, Avocados, Bananas (ripe), Berries, Carrots, Celery, Currants, Dates & figs (fresh), Garlic, Gooseberry, Grapes (less sweet), Grapefruit, Guavas, Herbs (leafy green), Lettuce (leafy green), Nectarine, Peaches (sweet), Pears (less sweet), Peas (fresh sweet), Persimmon, Pumpkin (sweet), Sea salt, Spinach	**6.0** Cigarette tobacco (roll your own), Cream of Wheat (unrefined), Fish, Fruit juices with sugar, Maple syrup (processed), Molasses (sulphured), Pickles (commercial), Breads (refined) of corn, oats, rice & rye, Cereals (refined) e.g. Weetabix, corn flakes, Shellfish, Wheat germ, Whole Wheat foods, Wine, Yogurt (sweetened)
7.5 Apples (sour), Bamboo shoots, Beans (fresh green), Beets, Bell Pepper, Broccoli, Cabbage, Cauliflower, Carob, Daikon, Ginger (fresh), Grapes (sour), Kale, Kohlrabi, Lettuce (pale green), Oranges, Parsnip, Peaches (less sweet), Peas (less sweet), Potatoes & skin, Pumpkin (less sweet), Raspberry, Sapote, Strawberry, Squash, Sweet corn (fresh), Tamari, Turnip, Vinegar (apple cider)	**6.5** Bananas (green), Buckwheat, Cheeses (sharp), Corn & rice breads, Egg whole (cooked hard), Ketchup, Mayonnaise, Oats, Pasta (whole grain), Pastry (wholegrain & honey), Peanuts, Potatoes (with no skins), Popcorn (with salt & butter), Rice (basmati), Rice (brown), Soy sauce (commercial), Tapioca, Wheat bread (sprouted organic)

The Answer to Cancer – An Electron Deficit Condition

Slightly Alkaline to Neutral pH 7.0	Slightly Acid to Neutral pH 7.0
7.0 Almonds, Artichokes (Jerusalem), Barley-Malt (sweetener-Bronner), Brown Rice Syrup, Brussel Sprouts, Cherries, Coconut (fresh), Cucumbers, Egg plant, Honey (raw), Leeks, Miso, Mushrooms, Okra, Olives ripe, Onions, Pickles (home-made), Radish, Sea salt, Spices, Taro, Tomatoes (sweet), Vinegar (sweet brown rice), Water Chestnut Amaranth, Artichoke (globe), Chestnuts (dry roasted), Egg yolks (soft cooked), Essene bread, Goat's milk and whey (raw), Horseradish, Mayonnaise (homemade), Millet, Olive oil, Quinoa, Rhubarb, Sesame seed (whole), Soy beans (dry), Soy cheese, Soy milk, Sprouted grains, Tempeh, Tofu, Tomatoes (less sweet), Yeast (nutritional flakes)	**7.0** Barley malt syrup, Barley, Bran, Cashews, Cereals (unrefined with honey-fruit-maple syrup), Cornmeal, Cranberries, Fructose, Honey (pasteurized), Lentils, Macadamias, Maple syrup (unprocessed), Milk (homogenized) and most processed dairy products, Molasses (unsulphered organic), Nutmeg, Mustard, Pistachios, Popcorn & butter (plain), Rice or wheat crackers (unrefined), Rye (grain), Rye bread (organic sprouted), Seeds (pumpkin & sunflower), Walnuts Blueberries, Brazil nuts, Butter (salted), Cheeses (mild & crumbly), Crackers (unrefined rye), Dried beans (mung, adzuki, pinto, kidney, garbanzo), Dry coconut, Egg whites, Goats milk (homogenized), Olives (pickled), Pecans, Plums, Prunes, Spelt

PART 3
HOW TO SLOW THE AGING PROCESS

Chapter 10
Appendix 1

MAGNETISM AND EARTHING.

The human body is made up of up to 90% water. This water has a high saline content which makes it a very good conductor of electricity and the cerebro-spinal fluid is made up of almost pure Vitamin C which is an extraordinarily good conductor of electrons. Finally, the brain is made up of totally unsaturated fatty proteins so that it behaves as an organic, body-temperature super conductor. There being no resistance to the passage of electromagnetic currents through its medium.

The whole structure of our bodies and particularly the brain-spine complex, act as a perfect biological antenna conducting fluctuations in the earth's electromagnetic field throughout the entire structure. These fluctuations have a major effect on our hormones and as far back as 1964, L. Gross showed that a small difference in a magnetic field can produce physical effects:-

Magnetic fields modify the way functions of electrons in macro-molecules, producing a greater paramagnetic susceptibility, which leads to a slow-down in reaction speed and the rate at which the RNA and DNA are synthesised.

In other words, the replication of DNA macro-molecules is mediated by the action of the fluctuation in the earth's magnetic field. DNA is very sensitive to magnetic fields and turns perpendicularly to a magnetic field.
Its electromagnetic sympathy is implicit in its structure and behaviour since it's a left-handed spiral form.

The earth's magnetic field has fluctuated over the millennia and these fluctuations have had a profound effect on humankind, particularly on our life span.

Dr. Okai of Kyorin University in Japan has discovered an increase in the life span of red blood cells in the bodies of mice and a strong magnetic field environment. Human beings are not mice but our metabolisms are very similar and Dr. Okai hypothesises that the substantial increase in longevity in his test subjects may be due to the sterilising action and other positive life prolonging attributes possessed by the magnetic field.

Magnetic fields on health.

Any conducting substance moving in the presence of a magnetic field generates electricity. Accordingly, the blood flow generates electricity which ionises the blood and as we're seeing when any molecule is ionised, it's very active. Accordingly, the magnetic field and your heart pumping energy force the separation of plus and minus ions and these active ions have been detected to loosen and chip away plaque and cholesterol build up in the arteries.

In its active stage, each ion has an electric field which induces water to be hexagonally structured and active. Consequently, the water content of the blood is extremely sensitive to fluctuations in the earth's magnetic field and throughout the billions of years of our evolution, it's axiomatic that our life expectancy has fluctuated in direct proportion to the strength of the earth's magnetic field.

Decline.

The earth's magnetic field has been measurably declining for the last 300 years and it is postulated by many leading scientists that we are now entering a period of time when the earth's polarity will reverse. This has happened many times throughout history and is usually a time of much chaos, strife, ill-health and systemic collapse.

At this point, it's worth the mention that on a personal level, you can strengthen your own exposure to the earth's magnetic field by wearing a small array of magnets.

These significantly improve your circulation and the quality of your blood in ionic terms as well as boosting the hormonal activity within your structure.

The wearing of a properly constructed magnetic device actually strengthens the electrical currents in your body. This is because any electrolyte (such as human blood) moving through a magnetic field will have a strengthened electrical potential.

By properly constructed, I mean that the device must be negative toward the body and positive away, since the flow of magnetic gauss is from positive to negative. In this way we put energy into the flow rather than taking it out.

Diurnal flow

As it circles the earth the moon "pumps" the ionosphere up and down as it pulls the tides around the planet. This has the effect of pumping the energy flow of electrons from the negative earth to the positive ionosphere and this pumping action causes the electrons to flow along the metabolic pathways of the body which are the energy lines of classical acupuncture.

Using an electron microscope, one can actually see electrons entering and exiting the skin at acupuncture points where they form a helical flow which helix or vortex directs the pressure of the electronic flow in and out of the body. This is known in Chinese medicine as the flow of "chi" or "prana" in the Hindu tradition. Human beings, and indeed all living creatures, are subjected to this energy flow and have a magnetic sensitivity which in man is centred on the pineal gland (the third eye) which sensitivity in large part affects the electromagnetic activity in their bodies. By insulating oneself from this flow of energy, one is shortening one's life and damaging one's health.

Our new electronic environment

These magnetic devices will provide a certain amount of enhanced protection to your system. However, there is much yet to be done in this direction as I will explain in a moment.

We depend on electricity for almost everything. We live in a world which is increasingly run and organised through electricity. This has given rise to a multitude of electrical machines which have become part of the fabric of our daily lives. The use of computers, televisions, central heating pumps, fluorescent lights, photocopiers, washing machines, radios and bedside lamps, plus a host of other equipment, have created a huge web of electrical wiring in every house, factory, public building and office. This complex new environment can have serious effects on our general health and well-being.

This is because the method of power generation used in almost every electrical device or system in use on the planet today is creating artificial spiral vortex fields at right angles to the current flow which rotate in the opposite direction to the ones which occur naturally and are used within living systems.

In the human system, rhythmic patterns of activity throughout the organism are of a left-handed nature, they are the result of the movement of force fields which initially organised amino acid/matter into left-handed structures. These left-handed forces, the product of a natural magnetic field, continue to operate in a healthy body. When they are subjected to interference from fields rotating in the opposite direction, a break down in the signals can occur. Aberrant signals emanating from an oscillator in a disturbed pattern can bring about profoundly different growth instructions in single cells and this is nowadays a major stressor which can lead to cancerous states in the body. This is because the cells are receiving the wrong growth instructions from the DNA (which a normal function has a left-hand rotation) which is being stimulated by the wrong signals.

How to protect yourself

It is vital to good health and particularly to longevity to learn now how to protect yourself against the modern mechanically driven electromagnetic environment.

The planet is a 6 sextillion metric ton battery that is constantly being replenished by solar radiation, lightning and heat from its molten core. The rhythmic pulsations of natural energy flowing through and from the surface of the earth to the protective shields of the Van Allen belt, keep the biological machinery of life on earth running in rhythm and balance.

Each living creature is a collection of dynamic electrical circuits and in the complexity of our bodies, trillions of cells constantly transmit and receive energy in the course of their programmed bio-chemical reactions.

Our hearts, brains, nervous systems, muscles and immune systems are prime examples of electrical systems operating within our bio-electrical body. In a study published in 2005 by electrical engineer Roger Applewhite, two significant factors were confirmed:-

1. Electrons move from the body to the earth and vice-versa when the body is grounded. The effect is sufficient to maintain the body at the same negative-charged potential as the earth.

2. Grounding dramatically reduces the impact of electromagnetic fields on the body.

The Applewhite study showed the protective effect of earthing against environmental electric fields and in his classic lectures on physics in the early 1960s, Nobel Prize physicist, Richard Feynman describes the earth's subtle energies.

The surface, as we have seen, has an abundance of electrons which give it a negative charge. If you're standing outside on a clear day wearing shoes or standing on an insulating surface, there is an electrical charge of some 350 volts between the earth and the top of your head if you're about 6 feet tall. That is to say, zero at ground level and 350 volts in the area of your head.

You don't get a shock because air is a relatively poor conductor and has virtually no electrical current flow.

If, on the other hand, you're standing outside in your bare feet, you are earthed, your whole body is in electrical contact with the earth's surface.

Your body is a relatively good conductor. Your skin and the earth's surface make a continuous charged surface at the same electrical potential. Therefore, any object in direct contact with the earth essentially becomes part of the earth and resides within the protective umbrella of the earth's natural electric field.

Accordingly, if you want to protect yourself from the worst effects of the modern mechanically driven electromagnetic environment, then it is important for you to walk barefoot on the earth for at least half an hour each day.

Earthing is dose related

The longer you are able to ground yourself in your daily life, the more stable, energetic and robust your body functions will be and the greater your ability to heal. The reason for this is that the human immune system evolved over millions of years. During this great span of time, we lived mostly in barefoot contact with the earth. We were naturally earthed. This meant that the biological clock of the body was continually calibrated by the pulse of the earth that governs the circadian rhythms of all life on the planet.

```
         SPHERICAL              MAGNETIC
          EARTH                   LINES
```

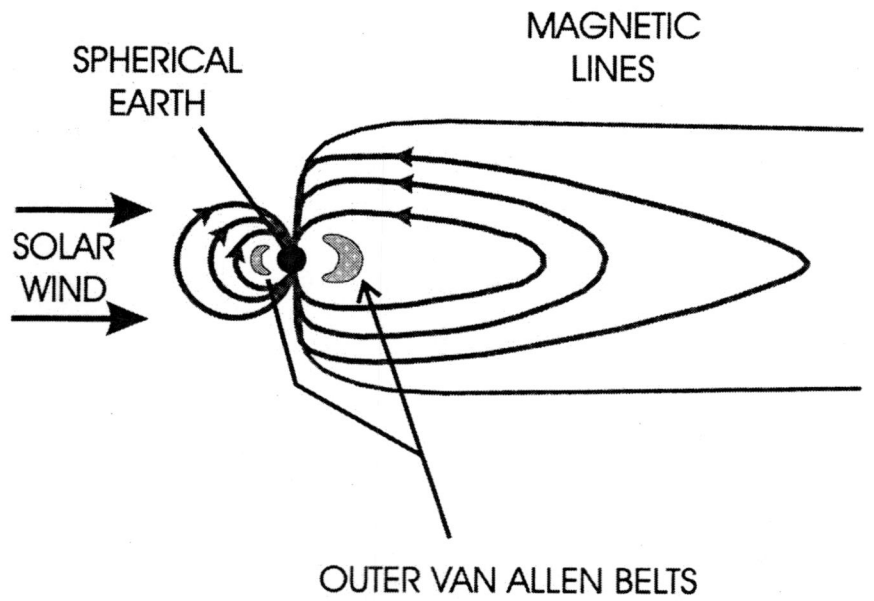

Earth's magnetic field

Disconnecting

What happens to the human body when it's separated from the subtle evolutionary signals from the earth was dramatically shown by experiments in Germany at the world famous Max Planck Institute during the 60s and 70s.

Researchers intentionally isolated volunteers for months at a time in underground rooms electrically shielded from the rhythms in the earth's electrical field. Patterns of body temperature, sleep, urinary excretion and other physiological activities were carefully monitored. All the participants developed a variety of abnormal or chaotic patterns. They experienced disturbed sleep and waking patterns, out of sync hormonal production and overall disruption in basic body regulation.

Whilst we don't live underground, as did these volunteers, we live above the ground and on the ground but we've disconnected ourselves from these bio-rhythms by wearing shoes.

The late Dr. William Rossi, a Massachusetts podiatrist and footwear industry historian, wrote in a 1999 article in Podiatry Management: "A natural gait is biomechanically impossible for any shoe wearing person, it took 4 million years to develop our unique human foot and our consequent distinctive form of gait – a remarkable feat of bio-engineering. Yet in only a thousand years and with one carelessly designed instrument, our shoes, we've warped the pure anatomical form of human gait, obstructing its engineering efficiency, afflicting it with strains and stresses and denying its natural grace of form and ease of movement head to foot".

He further wrote in Footwear News in 1997: "The Sole (or Plantar Surface of the Foot) is richly covered with some 1,300 nerve endings per square inch. That's more than found on any other part of the body of comparable size and is there to keep us in touch with the earth - the real physical world around us".

The paws of all animals are equally rich in nerve endings and the earth is covered with an electromagnetic layer from which every living thing including human beings draws energy.

The energy residing on the surface of the earth is primarily electrical and the central theme of this part of this paper is that we draw electrical energy through our feet in the form of free electrons fluctuating at many frequencies. These frequencies reset our biological clock and provide the body with electrical energy. The electrons themselves flow into the body, equalising and maintaining it at the electrical potential of the earth.

The original light weight soft sole, heelless and simple moccasin – a piece of crudely tanned leather that envelopes the foot and is fastened on with rawhide thongs – is possibly the closest we've ever come to an ideal shoe. It dates back more than 14,000 years.

To substantiate this, Dr. Morris Ghaly measured the circadian secretion of cortisol on people before and after they slept grounded over a period of a few weeks. The study was published in a 2004 issue of the Journal of Alternative and Complementary Medicine and the conclusion was:-

"Earthing during sleep resynchronises cortisol secretion more in alignment with its natural, normal rhythm – highest at 8am and lowest at midnight".

Whether you sleep grounded or walk barefoot on the earth, the effect of earthing out all of the unnatural energies impacting your body's antenna is profoundly beneficial.

<u>Blood Thinning</u>

Experiments conducted by Stephen Sinatra MD with a group of clinical physicians, PhD's working in the medical field, nurses and the author Clint Oba showed an astonishing effect on blood viscosity of grounding.

This experiment involved taking a drop of blood before and after 40 minutes of grounding by electro patches, and then examining the fresh unstained blood under a dark field microscope.

The after-grounding picture showed that people's blood dramatically changes within a short period of time after an individual is in contact with the earth. Specifically, there were considerably fewer formations of red blood cells associated with clamping and clotting. The blood appeared to be thinner.

The result suggested that individuals with heart disease and inflammatory thick blood (typical in cardiovascular disease and diabetes) may reap huge benefits from simply earthing themselves on a regular basis.

Inflammation and ageing

Inflammation comes in two forms, acute or chronic. The acute form takes place as an initial response to the body to harmful stimuli. It involves the mobilisation of plasma from the blood into the injured tissue and in the short-term this is a beneficial reaction.

On the other hand, chronic inflammation means a progressive shift in the type of activity going on at the site of the inflammation.

This occurs when you get simultaneous destruction and healing of the tissue, but also a harmful free-radical encroachment into healthy surrounding territory.

(Free radicals are the basis of chronic disease and the ageing process, particularly accelerated ageing and limited lifespan.)

This occurs when normal inflammation veers out of control because of the lost contact with the earth. People are suffering from an electron deficiency, that is to say not enough free electrons on hand to neutralise the rampaging free-radicals. Unfortunately, these go on to attack the adjacent healthy tissue in an ever expanding vicious cycle. The non-stop attack mode generates an auto-immune response manifesting as chronic inflammation and the immune system has run amuck. The pain generated in this process is entirely due to the positive free radical reactions and can be considerably assuaged by continually earthing the system/body on a regular basis.

Earthing then considerably benefits each and every one of us, reduces chronic pain, energises us, reduces or eliminates jet lag, dramatically speeds healing and helps prevent bed sores, lessens hormonal and menstrual problems, accelerates recovery from intense athletic activity, thins blood and improves blood pressure and flow. It normalises the body's biological rhythms, lowers stress and promotes calmness in the body by cooling down the nervous system and stress hormones. It improves sleep and protects the body against potentially health disturbing environmental electromagnetic forces.

To conclude, the wearing of magnetic bracelets and similar devices is highly beneficial as we have seen, as is the practice of earthing on a daily basis. It's now possible to buy special sandals which will earth you automatically and equally possible to buy bed sheets which either plug into earth systems in the house or can be attached to copper rods driven into the ground to earth your body and pick up the earth's natural rhythms whilst sleeping.

Magnetic field

During the last 500 years the Earth's magnetic-field strength has decreased by about 50% and Dr. Nakagawa of the Isuzu Hospital, Tokyo, Japan has written a thesis entitled: "Magnetic Field Deficiency Syndrome and Magnetic Treatment". In this thesis he points out and lists syndromes of modern people that he relates to magnetic field deficiency. Dr. Nakagawa believes that the current trend of the decreasing strength of the earth's magnetic field is creating magnetic field deficiency syndrome since he believes that there is a direct relationship between the decrease in the earth's magnetic field acting on the human body and the improvement of abnormal conditions of the human body by the application of magnetic fields.

Given that this is now a well-proven hypothesis in practice, it is then well worthwhile wearing a magnetic health device so as to preserve your internal electromagnetic environment and health.

Chapter 11

HOW TO LENGTHEN YOUR (HEALTHY) LIFE
Appendix 2

THE HUMAN ANTENNA

Our blood, as I've said, has the same composition as sea water of the Cambrian period. The same salts that are present in sea water are present in all of us as, is the same sensitivity to the oscillations of our surroundings to a greater or lesser degree. This has had a substantial bearing on our evolution. Evidence from magnetised rocks show that the earth's field strength has varied considerably in the past and this variation has had a considerable influence both on our behaviour and on our evolution.

Here's how

The magnetic fields of the moon and the sun plus the effects of the solar wind's magnetic field, induce a magnetic field in the earth of a strength depending on its mineral content, their relative distances, and the state of the intervening electrolyte, the air.

Since an electric current is induced in any conductor moving in a magnetic field, the mineral content of the conductor has a bearing on the degree of conductivity.

Humans are such a conductor moving in the earth's magnetic field and the current induced in our blood, by virtue of continuous movement, supplies oxygen to the lungs and tissues and most plentifully to the brain. The brain transmits energy to the nerves and muscles by means of electric impulses and so the strength of the magnetic field affects our response.

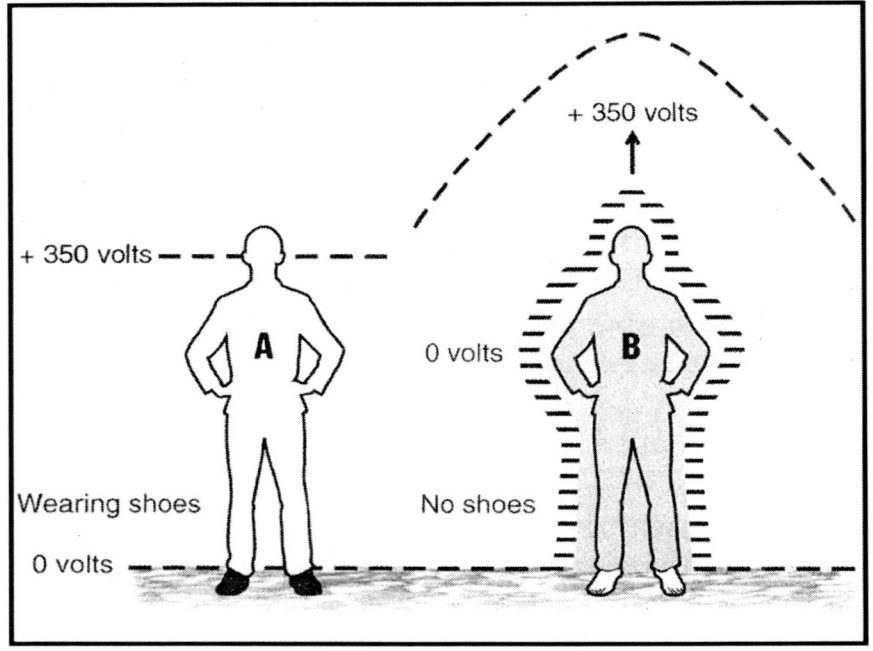

The Answer to Cancer – An Electron Deficit Condition

The 'umbrella' effects of earthing

Blood is conditioned by diet, exertion and the behaviour of the other organs in the body and is also liable, as a conductor in the earth's magnetic field, to changes in that field which may sometimes make it exceed or fall below its normal pH.

As we've seen earlier, alterations in the pH, which currently averages between 7.3 and 7.4, will produce corresponding changes in the activity of the brain and nervous system. Departure from the normal alkalinity of the blood, a change in pH, is well shown by nervous disturbances.

Increasing alkalinity leads to an excessive neuromuscular irritability which is known as tetany, preceded by headaches, nausea and mental confusion and also lassitude.

On the other hand, a failure to maintain alkalinity leads to extreme breathlessness, stupor and with terminal coma.

Ancient Civilisations

The peoples who built the great civilisations of the eras before the first millennium BC were differentiated from us by a physiological factor which influenced the conductivity of their bodies, so that changes which we can only detect by sensitive instruments when we are in normal health, were then perceptible by the brain.

The changes which have taken place in our physiology and behaviour over the millennia are directly linked to changes in the earth's electromagnetic field.

Such changes, no doubt, occurred very gradually by changes in the mineral content of man's blood and account for the cultural and anatomical changes detected by anthropologists in the history of mankind, dividing flint-users from copper, copper from bronze-using man and bronze from iron.

For example, the early Egyptian civilisation was based upon the use of copper, iron only being available from meteorite sources. The Egyptians recording something in the region of 14,000 years of practice in their religion seemed to be dominantly concerned with balancing, explaining and making allowances for man's changing levels of excitability brought about by the general anaemia in our species at that time.

The mineral content of a living creature is the most important component of their resistance to electrical stimuli. Since conductivity is a reciprocal of resistivity, it must be increased where resistivity is low. Resistance of the human body depends principally on the mineral content which is contained largely in the blood and bones. So, man's conductivity will be increased when his resistivity is low as it is in anaemia. Copper is a much better conductor than iron and far less retentive so that one might expect the metabolism of an anaemic person to be affected and his behaviour to be more impulsive and changeable, more susceptible to exogenous electrical rhythms such as those of the earth's field or of an artificial magnetic field.

As we've seen, there was very little iron in early Egypt but an abundance of copper. With the introduction of iron which is a constitution of haemoglobin and much more retentive than copper, there came about a profound change in human behaviour. Up to the introduction of iron across the board in human society, human kind was chiefly vegetarian and relatively anaemic. However, when the blood of our species became concentrated by the increase of protein, that is to say, by the consumption of much more meat in our diet, and further stabilised by the addition of iron, then sensitivity decreased, man became more independent of his environment, longevity fell away dramatically and society changed visibly.

Cro-Magnon

35,000 years BC in south-west Europe more or less in the shadow of the Pyrenees, the first and most enduring of all human civilisations existed and lasted for an astonishing 25,000 years.

This stone-age civilisation, created by the first really modern Europeans, was more long-lasting than any that had succeeded it. It was ten times longer than the reign of the Pharaohs in Egypt, 25 times longer than the thousand years of Greco-Roman history and extraordinarily durable.

Although the historical lineage of humankind stretches much further back (5 or 6 million years) it left nothing behind other than stone implements with which they broke open nuts and butchered what they had hunted.

The arrival of mankind in south-western Europe was the culmination of the great migrations, a hundred thousand years earlier, which caused modern Homo sapiens to leave his African homeland and spread outwards to every corner of the earth.

Cro-Magnon was the first to leave behind an image of his civilisation and back in those days we were great technical innovators. Whilst our predecessors' stone tools had scarcely changed in a million years, we invented the spear thrower, the harpoon, lamps to illuminate caves and drills that could put an eye in a needle, along with ropes to bind tents together.

This burst of creativity shows that Cro-Magnon was not simply an improved version of his early ancestors but was a totally unprecedented entity who inaugurated the first and most astonishing of all human civilisations.

Whereas, we have the knowledge and technology of earlier civilisations to draw upon, the genius of the Cro-Magnon is that they worked it all out for themselves. We know that the Sahara desert began to form around a hundred thousand years ago, and that large swaths of the northern African part of the continent began to dry out. This was probably the cause of the great diaspora of humankind from Africa, along the coastal byways to colonise the rest of the world. And we also know that this period of drying out was dependent entirely upon solar activity i.e. the greater intensity of the sun having the effect of drying out large areas of the habitable section of the globe. (By habitable section I mean those areas between the tropics of Cancer and Capricorn which were not then subjected to the ice age).

The rapid changes in our species brought about by the stressful necessity of migration may well be one of the causes of the sudden explosion of creativity in Cro-Magnon but, certainly up until that time and even beyond, humankind was still predominantly anaemic subsisting in the main on an alkaline diet.

With the coming of the various metal ages, mankind certainly became more excitable. This excitability brought about by an extreme sensitivity to fluctuations in the electromagnetic environment, clearly gave rise to various great religious imperatives at the heart of which is a desire to comprehend, regulate and ascribe power to the influences of the environment. At that time solar worship and lunar worship were dominant long before monotheism gained ground.

Iron

The introduction of iron on a large scale within human civilisation effected a profound turning point in human development since its ubiquity introduced high levels of haemoglobin into the blood of our species, which in turn made us more "down to earth" and much more aggressive.

This aggression stems from an alteration in the alkaline balance of the blood where a higher incidence of haemoglobin will mean that less oxygen is absorbed / available which causes the entire system to acidify.

Another factor which is cohort in this change is the fluctuations in the earth's magnetic field over this time.

The relationship between man's behaviour, his electro-chemical makeup and his environment are well grounded in science as we've seen and the explosion of our aggressive, short-lived species across the planet in recent millennia is largely due to the profound change in our nature which took place at the collapse of the Bronze Age when iron began to dominate our lives.

The simplest way to reduce the influence of iron on your bloodstream is to eat with bronze knives and forks, to plough the land or till the earth with hardened copper implements and to cook in copper or tin pots.

The reason for this is that minute quantities of iron scrape off steel eating utensils, are scoured off iron and steel cooking pots, thus entering our system. Equally, soil structure is reduced, in effect "shorted out", by the use of steel or iron gardening implements, ploughs and the like, the fertility of the soil being considerably enhanced by the use of copper. These are well known bio-dynamic remedies and they work.

Ultimately, what we are concerned with in seeking enhanced longevity is a more efficiently functioning human antenna. This because it is the steady rhythmic fluctuations in the planet's energy which entrain, stimulates and maintains life. Reduce the functioning of the antenna by bad diet etc. and you reduce your lifespan. Increase it and you increase your lifespan!

The human frame is a superb antenna being composed of about a fathom of salty water. This is an excellent electrolyte, in other words it carries and transmits the vast range of frequencies which surround us in this world. This outer electrolyte surrounds the spinal column and the spinal cord is made up of almost pure Vitamin C which, as we've seen from the earlier chapters, is a fantastic conductor.

On top of this accumulator/battery-like structure there sits a cranium in which resides a brain, once again a room temperature superconductor and this very housing, the skull, has a profound role to play in this antenna-like structure as we shall see.

Magnetic lines of force

The Earth has the properties of a large magnet and generates streams of magnetic energy that follow lines of force. If you turn on any motor or generator you can hear its energy at work since it will hum as it revolves. This hum is associated with the energy itself and not so much the movements of the rotor through the air. If the motor stalls while the power is turned on, the hum will become louder! The electrical and magnetic forces in the motor generate the sound waves. The earth itself acts as a giant dynamo and produces similar sound waves revolving as it does one revolution every 24 hours. The hum that the earth, acting as a dynamo, produces is at a very low frequency, a low vibration and thus it goes unnoticed as we go about our daily lives. It is our planet's inaudible fundamental pulse or rhythm.

There are a great many pulses and rhythms at work within this structure of the earth since any change in the density of an elastic medium can serve as a source for sound. The earth's energy includes mechanical, thermal, electrical, magnetic, nuclear, and chemical action, each a source of sound.

The most common sound waves are produced by the mechanical vibrations of solids, liquids and gases. Solid vibrators include strings and rods, membranes and plates, shells, bells and three dimensional extended objects like the earth itself.

Known as the Schumann resonances, there are fundamental vibrations which are the result of electrical activity between the earth and its upper atmospheric layers. Collectively known as electromagnetic cavity, the elements that make it up are the earth, the ionosphere, the troposphere and the magnetosphere. The fundamental frequency of the vibrations is calculated to be 7.83 hertz with overlaying frequencies of 14, 20, 26, 32, 37 and 43 hertz.

Chapter 12

Resonance and Harmonics

Most of these sound frequencies are well below our levels of hearing, but nevertheless have a profound effect on our lives, our emotions and our energy levels.

Their energies resonate within us and indeed we are formed of harmonic structures which are the basis of these resonances.

To understand resonance, it's best to use the analogy of a piano.

Press down a key or several keys forming a chord, without actually striking the note, then un-damp the strings by pressing the loud pedal. Play the corresponding note on an octave higher and the strings you have opened on the lower octave will vibrate in sympathy. If you hum into the piano in the same pitch, the strings will again respond. This transfer of energy is due to resonance. The transmission of energy and vibration go hand in hand. The strings of a musical instrument are induced to vibrate, and the energy reaches our ears in the form of sound waves.

When airborne sound forces mechanical vibrations in several piano strings that vibrate at different frequencies, the phenomenon known as harmonics is at work. Elements will absorb energy from a source more efficiently if they're of the same frequency. Multiples of the fundamental forcing frequency, known as harmonic frequencies, will also efficiently absorb this energy and vibrate in their natural resonance.

This is why soldiers are instructed to break step when marching across a bridge because each step of an individual soldier acts as a force on the bridge. If the rest of the company joins this soldier in marching together across the bridge, the energy provided by that one step is amplified many times over and the bridge will vibrate in time to the march.

The pounding of feet on the bridge is known as the forcing frequency and if this frequency happens to coincide with the natural frequency at which the bridge resonates, the absorption of energy will be maximised and the vibration of the bridge will become much greater up to the point where it can shake itself apart. This is explained in the Encyclopaedia Britannica:-

If the damping is very small, a vibrator will draw correspondingly large average power from the source, especially resonance. If the damping becomes effectively zero or even negative, as can happen under certain peculiar circumstances, the power withdrawal may become so great as to lead to a runaway vibration that may destroy the vibrator.

A coupled oscillator

The human body when earthed (i.e. in its bare feet) forms a coupled oscillator that is in harmonic resonance with the earth. A coupled oscillator is an object that is in harmonic resonance with another, usually larger vibrating object. When set into motion, the coupled oscillator will draw energy from the source and vibrate in sympathy as long as the source continues to vibrate.

It's been known for some time that vibrations at around 6 hertz influence the brain and produce various effects in humans and we now know in fact that the brain frequencies entrain with the Schumann resonances across their full spectrum.

NASA consultant and acoustic engineer, Tom Danley, has identified four frequencies which form an F sharp chord which is said to be the harmonic of our planet. And in the same way that a bell is tuned to a fundamental hum and its harmonics removed by removing metal from the critical areas, these low volume frequencies are the forcing frequencies which have shaped mankind's development into the species that we are today. (More of which later).

To bring things to a head!

The human skull could be described as being generally round with an aperture on one face, is connected to the spine which we've already seen is a superb transmitter of information received throughout the body. The human skull is fundamentally a Helmholtz resonator which responds to vibrations and actually maximises the transfer of energy from the source of the vibrations. A resonator is normally made out of metal but it can be made out of any other materials and a classic example of a Helmholtz resonator is a hollow sphere with a round opening that is one-tenth to one-fifth the diameter of the sphere.

The size of the sphere determines the frequency at which it will resonate. If the resonant frequency of the resonator is in harmony with the vibrating source, such as a tuning fork, it will draw energy from the fork and resonate and at a greater amplitude than the fork is able to do without its presence. In other words, it forces the fork to greater energy output than what is normal, or "loads" the fork. Unless the energy in the fork is replenished, its energy will be exhausted quicker than it normally would be without the Helmholtz resonator. But as long as the source continues to vibrate, the resonator will continue to draw energy from it. Thus we regard the ever vibrating earth as the resonator and the human structure as the antenna/Helmholtz resonator we can see that energies emanating from the ever vibrating planet are drawn in and utilised by the human form both as a source of energy and structural arbiter.

By way of reinforcing what I'm saying here, I point to the fact that human babies put on an initial spurt of growth after their birth and put on weight well in excess of the amount of food that they take in.

Further yet, astronauts and also people confined in nuclear submarines for great lengths of time, both groups exhibit disorientation, loss of bone growth and general deterioration until returned to the normal surface environment.

In his classic text, "The Geomagnetic Field and Life" by the Russian scientist Alexander Dubrov, Professor Dubrov combines western studies with extensive research in eastern Europe over the last 20-odd years and provides general support for the field and resonance concepts of this work. He regards the moment at which an organism begins to grow, and the specific interaction of genetic and molecular polarities with a geomagnetic field, as of fundamental importance to its future development. The geomagnetic forces are essentially life-giving, while the complementary gravitational forces stabilise these effects.

If we think of genes not as static on-off groups of chemicals, but as oscillators with coherent frequency properties, then there's no inherent theoretical problem about embryonic growth. An ordered set of oscillators will produce a consistent patterning of material. It will ensure that the formation of new structures will occur according to definite time sequence. It will create patterns of rhythmic activity throughout the organism. It can account for degeneration and ageing as well as the initial growth patterns. It can explain in principle both the cell formation and the whole body formation.

There is now considerable experimental evidence that the geomagnetic field modifies genes and chromosomes (there is for instance a gene mutation of the insect Adalia which changes the wing colour from red to black and which changes correlate quite closely with the geomagnetic field. In versions of the X-chromosomes of the fruit fly have been shown to follow geo-magnetic field fluctuations). We now know that low frequency fields can affect mental states, physiological functions, bone structure, general patterning processes and germ plasma. These fields or vibrations directly affect a larger structure like the cell membrane which has unusual electromagnetic properties and also relate to unusual water structures in the cell membrane, these being sensitive to low frequency fields.

Summary

Our species development, health and lifespan are modulated and moderated by the geomagnetic field which expresses all the rhythms of vibration which derive from a very active planet. Thus, we are creatures intended by a life force to be in harmony with our planet and in order to be in harmony it is necessary to have as clean and properly functioning an antenna as possible.

It is also essential to keep in close touch with the planet's fundamental forcing frequencies, and to have mind to these as constants in our lives which affect the length of our lives.

The phrases we use in everyday language such as being off-key, off-colour, in-tune, keyed-up and so forth present our basic understanding of the forces which bear upon us and which formed us. Yet, as a species we have diverged far from our healthy bond with our environment, the consequence of this is that we reap the bitter harvest of a foreshortened life.

Addendum:

There is a hidden and little known cause of cancer which I've not included in this book. The reason for this is that it derives from knowledge that can only be imparted in person. It has to be learned, demonstrated and practiced before it becomes useful.

I teach this skill on my residential seminars which I run twice a year over a two-day period in a central location.

For further information and to register your interest in attending a seminar, please go to my website

www.keithfoster.co.uk

The Answer to Cancer – An Electron Deficit Condition

Further recommended reading list

Additional books by the author Keith Foster, FLS

1. *The Wisdom Way;* ISBN 978-0-9532407-9-1

2. *Harmonic Power Parts II – VI;* ISBN 978-0-9532407-7-7.

3. *Lifelight – (How to protect yourself from cancer or help yourself if you get ill).* ISBN 978-0 9532407-1-5

----

4. Foster, Paula FLS, *Practical Immunology – A New Healing Paradigm* ISBN 978-0-9532407-4-6

5. Green, Gerald *Breaking Through the Untouchable Diseases* ISBN 978-0-9532407-8-4

All of the above books are available via
www.keithfoster.co.uk

References / Sources

Nobel laureates

1   PAULING Dr. Linus. Twice Nobel Prize winner 1980's. *The role of Vitamin C as a powerful anti-cholesterol agent.*

2   SZENT-GYORGYI Albert. Discovered Vitamin C in 1932 and recommended use of Iodine. He received the Nobel Prize in Medicine in 1937.

3   WARBURG Otto, MD. Nobel Prize 1931 – *Research on respiratory enzymes certain vitamins and minerals that the body require for the utilization of oxygen in the cells.*

Other Sources

1. APPLEWHITE Roger. Electrical Engineer. *The effect of Grounding reduces Impact of EM Fields on Body.*

2. BATMANGHELIDJ Dr F. *Your Bodies Many Cries for Water* ISBN 978-0970245885

3. BECKER Robert O. MD and Gary Selden. *The Body Electric* ISBN 0-688-06971-1.

4. BROWNSTEIN Dr David M.D. *Iodine and Why You Need It.* ISBN 978-0-9660882-3-6

5. CAMERON Ewan and Linus Pauling *Cancer and Vitamin C* ISBN 0-446-97735-7.

6. CHERASKIN Dr Emanuel. Dr W. Marshall, Dr Ringsdorf Jr., and Dr Emily L. Sisley. *The Vitamin C Connection.* ISBN 0-7225-0908-1.

7. CLINTON Ober and Stephen T. Sinatra M.D. *Earthing.*
ISBN 978-1-59120-283-7

8. DANLEY Tom. NASA Consultant and Acoustic Engineer, has identified 4 frequencies which form an F# chord Encyclopaedia Britannica – *Definition of Power Function in Resonance.*

9. DAY Phillip. *Cancer* ISBN 0-9535012-4-8.

10. DICKENSON Donald, PhD. *How to Fortify your Immune System* ISBN 0-85140-633-5.

11. DOLL Sir Richard. (1977), *Stressed role of diet in cancer.* (Eminent British cancer specialist).

12. DUBROV Prof. Alexander. Russian Scientist. Confirms support for Field and Resonance Concepts.

13. DURRANT-PEATFIELD Dr Barry, MBBS LRCP MRCS. Medical advisor to Thyroid UK . *Fluoride and its effects on the thyroid production of hormones controlling appetite.*

14. EVANS John. *Mind Body and Electromagnetism*
ISBN 1-874498-00-8.

15. FEYNMAN Richard. Nobel Prize Physicist (1965) describes earth's subtle energies.

16. FOSTER Keith, FLS. *Harmonic Power Parts II – VI* (Sagax Publishing 2015) ISBN 978-0-9532407-7-0.

17. FRASSETTO Dr Lynda. (1996) University of California, San Francisco. Paper on *Bicarbonate levels in human blood vary with age.*

18. FULLER Buckminster, Architect. Carbon fullerenes are named after the Geodesic Dome he designed.

19. GHALY Dr Morris. (2004) Journal of Complementary Medicine. *Earthing During Sleep Resynchronises Cortisol Secretion During Sleep.* ISBN 978-0-9660882-3-6.

20. GROSS L. (1964). *Biological Effects of Magnetic Fields*, Vol. 1, Plenum Press, New York

21. LEVENSON Dr Frederick B. *The Causes and Prevention of Cancer* ISBN 0-283-99247-6.

22. McCance & Widdowson *The Composition of Foods*, 1978 – 2002.

23. NAKAGAWA Dr. The Isuzu Hospital, Tokyo, Japan *"Magnetic Field Deficiency Syndrome and Magnetic Treatment"*

24. NEWBOLD H.L. MD. *Vitamin C Against Cancer* ISBN 0-8128-6098-5.

25. OKAI Dr Kyorin. University, Japan. *Life Prolonging Attributes of Magnetic Fields.*

26. PESKIN Professor Brian Scott,. Texas Southern University, Dept. of Pharmacy & Health Sciences 1998-99. Co-author with clinical researcher Amid Habib, MD FAAP FACE . *The Hidden story of Cancer - Nutrition Solutions* (Pinnacle Press 2006).

27. ROSS Dr William. (1999) Article in Podiatry Management against wearing shoes. Also (1997) Footwear News. *Study of nerve endings on foot.*

28. SIMONCINI Dr T. Oncologist, *Cancer is a Fungus: A Revolution in Tumor Therapy* ISBN 88-87241-08-2.

29. SIRCUS Dr. Mark. *Sodium Bicarbonate – Natures Unique First Aid Remedy.* ISBN 978-0-7570-0394-3.

30. SOYKA Fred with Alan Edmonds, *The Ion Effect* ISBN 0-553-12866-3.

31. STONE Dr Irwin. (published in 1980's) *"Scurvy" the most misunderstood epidemic disease in the 20th century.*

32. STONE I. *The genetics of scurvy and the cancer problem.* J. Orthomolecular Psychiatry Vol 5, No. 3, 183-190, 1976.

33. VERKEEK Dr R. BSc MSc DIC PHD, Executive and Scientific Director, The Alliance for Natural Health. *The Pros and Cons of water chlorination.*

34. British Medical Journal 24thMarch 2006. Reviewing 96 trials including 44 with supplements and with ALA (alpha linoleic acid) from plants; the remainder being fish oils, found no evidence to a clear benefit from Omega 3 fats on health.

35. British Medical Journal, 7th April 2005; BMJ 2005;330:853 *No Sweet Surrender,* (article on sugar).

36. Canadian Journal of Surgery (1993); *Iodine relieves symptoms of fibrocystic breast disease in 70% of patients.*

37. The Cambridge International Institute for Medical Science. Paper on *Omega-3 and Omega-6 also fish oils.*

38. US Food & Drug Admin, Dept. of Health & Human Resources, FDA, Poisonous Plant Database, March 2006 Revision. 288 *Records of Soy*